No Carbs No Sugar Diet Plan

A Beginner's Step-by-Step Guide with Recipes and a Meal Plan

copyright © 2020 Bruce Ackerberg

All rights reserved No part of this book may be reproduced, or stored in a retrieval system, or transmitted in any form or by any means, electronic, mechanical, photocopying, recording, or otherwise, without express written permission of the publisher.

Disclaimer

By reading this disclaimer, you are accepting the terms of the disclaimer in full. If you disagree with this disclaimer, please do not read the guide.

All of the content within this guide is provided for informational and educational purposes only, and should not be accepted as independent medical or other professional advice. The author is not a doctor, physician, nurse, mental health provider, or registered nutritionist/dietician. Therefore, using and reading this guide does not establish any form of a physician-patient relationship.

Always consult with a physician or another qualified health provider with any issues or questions you might have regarding any sort of medical condition. Do not ever disregard any qualified professional medical advice or delay seeking that advice because of anything you have read in this guide. The information in this guide is not intended to be any sort of medical advice and should not be used in lieu of any medical advice by a licensed and qualified medical professional.

The information in this guide has been compiled from a variety of known sources. However, the author cannot attest to or guarantee the accuracy of each source and thus should not be held liable for any errors or omissions.

You acknowledge that the publisher of this guide will not be held liable for any loss or damage of any kind incurred as a result of this guide or the reliance on any information provided within this guide. You acknowledge and agree that you assume all risk and responsibility for any action you undertake in response to the information in this guide.

Using this guide does not guarantee any particular result (e.g., weight loss or a cure). By reading this guide, you acknowledge that there are no guarantees to any specific outcome or results you can expect.

All product names, diet plans, or names used in this guide are for identification purposes only and are the property of their respective owners. The use of these names does not imply endorsement. All other trademarks cited herein are the property of their respective owners.

Where applicable, this guide is not intended to be a substitute for the original work of this diet plan and is, at most, a supplement to the original work for this diet plan and never a direct substitute. This guide is a personal expression of the facts of that diet plan.

Where applicable, persons shown in the cover images are stock photography models and the publisher has obtained the rights to use the images through license agreements with third-party stock image companies.

Table of Contents

Introduction   7
The Need-to-Knows   10
   On carbohydrates   10
   On sugar   12
Understanding Insulin, Glucose, and Blood Sugar Basics   14
   What Happens When You Eat Sugar or Carbs   14
   How Glucose Enters the Bloodstream and Triggers Insulin   15
   What Insulin Actually Does   16
   Why Blood Sugar Swings Make You Tired, Moody, or Hungry   18
   How a No-Carb/No-Sugar Diet Interrupts This Cycle   20
The Health Risks of High-Carb and High-Sugar Consumption   24
   The Benefits of a No-Carb/No-Sugar Diet   27
   The Cons of a No-Carb/No-Sugar Diet   28
Common Myths about This Diet   31
   Myth 1: You Must Eliminate All Fruits   31
   Myth 2: This Is Just Another Fad Diet   32
   Myth 3: You'll Always Feel Weak or Tired   32
   Myth 4: You Can't Enjoy Food Anymore   33
   Myth 5: If You Cheat Once, You Ruin Everything   34
Preparing Yourself for the Diet   36
Learning How to Read Food Labels   40
Focusing on the Right Foods   43
Suggested Menu   45
   Low-carb oatmeal substitutes for breakfast or snacks   49
Food to Stay Away From   52
Foods to Eat More   54
Understanding Sugar Cravings: What Your Body Is Really Telling You   60

Biological Reasons You Crave Sugar	60
Emotional Triggers & Habits	63
What to Do Instead of Giving In to Sugar Cravings	67
Herbal or Supplement Support for Cravings	73
Curated Recipes	**75**
Grilled Lamb	76
Avocado and Smoked Salmon on a Slice of No-Carb Bread	78
Roasted Veggies	79
Ground Beef Stroganoff	80
Banana Bread	81
Chicken breasts and Garlic Spinach	83
Healthy Green Smoothie	85
Red Velvet Molten Lava Cake	86
Grilled Steak and Asparagus	88
Chicken Masala Crockpot Style	89
Broccoli and Tomato Salad with Nuts and Seeds	91
Balsamic-Glazed Chicken Thighs	92
Zero Carb Buttery Noodles	93
Zero Carb Bread	94
Zero Carb Pizza Crust	95
Zero Carb Breaded Tilapia	97
Baked Chicken Breasts	98
Baked Salmon	100
Baked Turkey Wings	102
Conclusion	**103**
FAQs and Troubleshooting	**105**
References and Helpful Links	**108**

Introduction

In recent years, more and more people have been embracing the idea of a no-carb, no-sugar diet as a way to lose weight and improve their overall health and well-being. While cutting out two major macronutrients can offer some potential benefits, it's important to understand not only what this type of diet entails but also the potential risks associated with it.

In this guide, we'll discuss what a no-carb, no-sugar diet is and its various benefits - from weight loss to improved mental clarity. We'll also take a look at the possible downsides of strictly eliminating these two macronutrients including nutrient deficiencies or digestive issues as well as provide tips for making sure that one is getting all the essential vitamins & minerals in their diet if they choose to go down this path.

To begin with, it's important to note that carbohydrates and sugars play an essential role in our body's energy production; without them, we would be unable to access quick bursts of energy when needed, especially if engaging in intense physical activity throughout the day. Furthermore, both simple (refined) sugars, as well as complex starches, can provide us with valuable nutrients like antioxidants, fibers, and other vitamins & minerals depending on what foods are being consumed within each group. Therefore, while cutting out these two food groups completely may lead to short-term gains such as initial weight loss, the long-term consequences can be quite drastic if other sources of adequate nutrition aren't found elsewhere within one's diet.

In addition to understanding how carbs & sugar function in our bodies and the risks associated with eliminating them from our regular meals, learning about which foods count towards each category is also vital for successfully following a no-carb/no-sugar eating plan. Different types of grains & flours contain varying amounts of both carbs & sugar so reading food labels carefully or doing research ahead of time can save someone from inadvertently "breaking" their own rules by consuming hidden sources hidden on ingredient lists!

We'll dive deeper into all these topics in upcoming posts so stay tuned for more information about going on a no-carb/no-sugar diet - its pros and cons, tips for success, and more!

In this step-by-step guide, you will be introduced to:

- The need-to-know about the no-carb, no-sugar diet
- The difference between healthy sugar and added sugar
- Suggestions to help yourself pace before starting the diet

- Identifying harmful labels on food
- What foods to eat and what foods to avoid
- Suggested recipes for food to eat within the diet
- Common mistakes to avoid

Going full-on in no-carb and no-sugar is not for everyone. However, it is for people who are willing to try a different kind of diet that may help them achieve their weight goals and lower their blood sugar levels. This guide will give you a lot of food options that will make the diet more bearable, especially for those who are beginners in the no-carb diet or no-sugar diet.

The Need-to-Knows

No-sugar, no-carb diet. A very terrifying suggestion. What could that possibly accomplish apart from giving dieters agonizing days? We have heard of low-carb, low-sugar diets.

A no-carb no-sugar diet is an eating plan that eliminates all sources of carbohydrates and sugars from the diet. This type of diet has become popular in recent years with some people claiming it helps with weight loss, energy levels, and overall health.

On carbohydrates

Carbohydrates are one of the three macronutrients and are essential for providing energy to our bodies. They are found in many different types of foods and come in many different forms. Carbohydrates can be categorized into two main groups: simple carbohydrates and complex carbohydrates.

Simple carbohydrates, or sugars, include items such as honey, fruit juice, candy, and table sugar. These typically provide quick sources of energy but may lead to sharp spikes in blood glucose levels if consumed in excess due to their easily digestible nature. On the other hand, complex carbohydrates contain longer chains of glucose molecules which take more time to break down in the digestive system leading to a slower release of glucose into the bloodstream and resulting in steadier energy levels throughout the day. Examples of complex carbohydrates include whole wheat bread and pasta, oats, beans, lentils, and quinoa among others.

In terms of health effects, both types of carbohydrates play an important role in our diets when consumed in moderation. Simple carbs can provide a boost of energy when needed while still being lower on the glycemic index than some processed foods like white bread or chips; this means they don't cause blood sugar levels to spike as quickly as these items do.

Complex carbs also have several benefits; they help keep us full for longer periods due to their higher fiber content which can help with weight management goals while also providing us with sustained energy throughout our days rather than short bursts followed by crashes that we might get from consuming too much sugar or processed foods.

Carbohydrates can be found naturally occurring in plant-based foods like fruits & vegetables as well as grains such as quinoa & rice; they may also be added to manufactured goods such as cereals & snacks during processing so it is always important to read labels before making any purchases! Additionally, some dairy products like milk & yogurt also naturally contain a small number of carbohydrates due to their lactose content.

On sugar

Added sugar is the main culprit of abandoned diets. People just can't get away from it. Even those who are trying to consciously steer away from sugar overlook their existence even on food that they think is not sweet, like condiments, crackers, tomato sauce, and even salad dressings. An average American consumes about 22 teaspoons of added sugar a day. Most of these are from the consumption of processed and prepared food.

There are two categories of sugar found in the foods we eat: naturally occurring sugars and added sugars. Naturally occurring sugars are present in foods in their natural state. Examples of these sources include fruits, vegetables, sugar cane, and sugar beets. Fructose is a natural sugar found in fruits, root vegetables, and honey. Lactose is present in dairy products such as milk and cheese. Sucrose is derived from sugar cane or sugar beets.

On the other hand, added sugars include any caloric sweeteners added to foods during processing or preparation. Major sources of added sugars are sodas, candies, cookies, fruit drinks, and dairy desserts.

The American Heart Association has recommended that Americans cut back on added sugar to prevent obesity and heart diseases. Excessive sugar consumption has been linked to other harmful conditions like high cholesterol, chronic inflammation, nonalcoholic fatty liver disease, and dental plaques and cavities.

There is no nutritional benefit from added sugar. Added sugars contribute zero nutrients to the food we eat. This is why they are usually labeled as empty calories. Despite this, added sugar is found in practically most of the items we find in grocery stores. Looking at the food labels, added sugars disguise themselves as different forms of sweeteners such as dextrose, maple syrup, or cane sugar. It is important to know their names to avoid adding them to the grocery list.

Understanding Insulin, Glucose, and Blood Sugar Basics

Insulin, glucose, and blood sugar are terms that we may often hear when it comes to discussing our health and nutrition. However, not many people understand the role they play in our body and how they affect our overall well-being.

What Happens When You Eat Sugar or Carbs

When you eat foods containing sugar or carbohydrates, your body begins to break them down during digestion. Carbohydrates, whether from bread, pasta, fruits, or veggies, eventually turn into a type of sugar called glucose. Glucose is your body's main source of energy, kind of like fuel for a car.

Once glucose is broken down, it enters your bloodstream. This is what people mean when they talk about "blood sugar." The amount of glucose in your blood rises after eating, depending on how much and what type of carbs you consumed.

How Glucose Enters the Bloodstream and Triggers Insulin

When you eat a meal, carbohydrates are broken down into glucose, which then enters your bloodstream. This causes your blood sugar levels to rise, and your body quickly recognizes this increase. To regulate these levels, the pancreas releases insulin, a hormone that acts like a key to "unlock" cells in your muscles, liver, and fat tissues. Once the cells are unlocked, they can absorb glucose, either to use immediately as energy or to store it for later needs, such as during periods of fasting or physical activity.

This process is essential for maintaining the body's energy balance. Your body is highly sensitive to keeping blood sugar levels within a healthy range. If blood sugar stays too high for an extended period, it can lead to issues like oxidative stress, inflammation, or even damage to vital organs such as the kidneys, heart, and eyes. Insulin plays a crucial role in preventing these problems by ensuring that glucose is swiftly removed from the bloodstream and directed into the cells where it's needed.

This intricate process helps maintain overall health and prevents complications associated with prolonged high blood sugar, such as diabetes. Understanding how this system works highlights the importance of a balanced diet and healthy lifestyle choices in supporting your body's natural processes.

What Insulin Actually Does

Insulin is a powerful hormone that acts like your body's conductor, keeping things running smoothly. While we've talked about how insulin helps regulate blood sugar, it also has a major role in how your body handles fat. Understanding this can help explain why balancing insulin levels is so important for health and weight management.

Unlocking Fat Storage Mode

When insulin levels are high, your body gets a signal that there's plenty of energy available from the glucose in your blood. Because of this, it shifts gears and starts storing that energy for later. This stored energy is primarily kept in the form of fat. Essentially, insulin unlocks your body's fat storage mode.

This process is completely normal and even necessary for survival. Your body is designed to store extra energy so it can have reserves for times when food isn't readily available. The challenge arises when insulin levels stay high for too long or too often because of consistently eating too many carbs or sugary foods. When this happens, more energy is stored as fat over time, and it becomes harder to lose weight.

Preventing Fat-Burning While Elevated

When insulin is elevated, your body focuses on storing energy, which means it stops burning fat for fuel. Think of it like this: if glucose is the fuel your body has in abundance after eating, insulin sends the message to "burn what's available now and save the fat for later." While this works well in the short term, it also means that as long as insulin levels remain high, your body won't tap into its fat reserves for energy.

This is one reason why stable insulin levels are so important. If your body is always busy storing energy and never given the chance to burn fat, it can lead to weight gain and other metabolic issues. Creating periods where insulin levels drop (like in between meals or during low-carb eating) allows your body to shift gears and use stored fat for energy.

Insulin's dual role in managing blood sugar and fat storage makes it a key player in your overall health. If insulin is constantly elevated due to high-carb or high-sugar diets, it encourages fat storage and limits your ability to burn fat. On the other hand, stabilizing insulin levels with balanced eating habits can support weight management and metabolic health.

By understanding how insulin works, you can make choices that help your body find balance. Focusing on whole, nutrient-dense foods and giving your body breaks between meals can help maintain steady insulin levels, allowing your natural fat-burning processes to work more effectively.

Why Blood Sugar Swings Make You Tired, Moody, or Hungry

Blood sugar levels play a crucial role in your energy, mood, and hunger throughout the day. When blood sugar rises and falls rapidly, this instability can lead to a range of physical and emotional effects. A key part of this process is what's commonly referred to as the "sugar crash" cycle. Here's a closer look at what happens in your body during this cycle and how it influences your overall well-being.

The "Sugar Crash"

Problems arise when blood sugar spikes too quickly, often after consuming foods high in sugar or refined carbohydrates like candy, pastries, or sugary drinks. These foods are broken down rapidly by your body, causing a quick surge of glucose into your bloodstream.

This rapid spike is followed by an equally sudden drop as your body responds by producing a large amount of insulin, a hormone that helps regulate blood sugar levels. Insulin works to bring blood sugar back down, but this sharp decline can result in what's commonly referred to as a "sugar crash."

During a sugar crash, your body struggles to maintain balance, leaving you feeling drained and out of sorts. This can manifest as fatigue, irritability, shakiness, or difficulty concentrating. Your brain, which relies on steady glucose levels for energy, may interpret the sudden drop as an energy shortage. In response, it triggers hunger signals and cravings, often for more sugary or carb-heavy foods, perpetuating the cycle.

Over time, frequent sugar spikes and crashes can strain your body and impact your overall energy stability, making it important to opt for more balanced, nutrient-dense meals that maintain steady blood sugar levels.

How Blood Sugar Swings Affect Energy

Rapid changes in blood sugar can leave you feeling like your energy levels are on a rollercoaster. After the initial burst of energy from a blood sugar rise, the subsequent crash can leave you feeling drained. If you rely on sugary snacks or refined carbs to quickly regain energy, you may unintentionally repeat the cycle throughout the day, leading to persistent fatigue.

Impacts on Mood

Blood sugar doesn't just impact your energy; it also affects your mood. Your brain relies on a steady supply of glucose to function properly. When blood sugar suddenly drops, your brain experiences a temporary loss of its primary fuel source, leading to irritability, difficulty concentrating, and moodiness.

This connection between blood sugar and mood is why people often feel short-tempered or overly emotional during a sugar crash. These effects can be even more noticeable if you're experiencing prolonged or frequent blood sugar swings.

Why You Feel Hungry

A sugar crash can also leave you feeling hungry, even if you've eaten recently. When blood sugar drops quickly, your body signals that it needs more fuel. This often leads to cravings for sugary or high-carb foods, since these provide a quick but short-lived energy boost.

Unfortunately, giving in to these cravings can perpetuate the cycle by causing another blood sugar spike, followed by another crash.

By understanding the sugar crash cycle and taking steps to prevent significant blood sugar swings, you can support more consistent energy levels, improved mood, and better appetite control throughout the day.

How a No-Carb/No-Sugar Diet Interrupts This Cycle

A no-carb or no-sugar diet can have a significant impact on your body's energy regulation and appetite control. By cutting out carbohydrates and sugars, these diets help to interrupt the cycle of rapid blood sugar fluctuations and insulin spikes. Here's how this approach works and why it can lead to more stable energy levels and improved appetite regulation.

Reducing Insulin Spikes

When you consume carbohydrates, your body breaks them down into glucose, which enters your bloodstream. A spike in blood sugar triggers your pancreas to release insulin, a hormone that helps move glucose into your cells for energy or storage. Eating sugary or refined carb-heavy foods causes blood sugar and insulin levels to rise sharply, often followed by a steep fall, leading to the "sugar crash."

A no-carb or no-sugar diet minimizes these effects by removing foods that cause rapid rises in blood sugar. Without the spikes in glucose levels, insulin production remains controlled and steady. This means your body avoids the extremes of high and low blood sugar that can contribute to feelings of fatigue, irritability, and sudden hunger.

Stabilizing Energy Levels

One of the major benefits of reducing or eliminating carbs and sugar is the stabilization of energy throughout the day. When blood sugar remains constant, your body doesn't experience the sharp peaks and dips that leave you feeling energetic one moment and drained the next. Instead, your energy comes from other sources, like fats, which are broken down more slowly and provide a steady supply of fuel.

People following low- or no-carb diets often report fewer mid-afternoon crashes and an overall sense of sustained energy. This happens because the body transitions to burning fat for fuel in a process known as ketosis, where energy is derived from fats rather than rapidly fluctuating glucose levels.

Managing Appetite

Blood sugar swings also affect hunger and cravings. When blood sugar drops after a spike, your body signals hunger, even if you've recently eaten. This is one reason why carb-heavy meals or snacks can lead to frequent hunger or overeating.

By removing the sharp rises and falls in blood sugar, a no-carb or no-sugar diet helps regulate your appetite more naturally. The consistent energy supply keeps hunger signals steady, reducing the intense cravings for quick-fix carb-rich foods. Additionally, high-fat and protein-based meals contribute to a feeling of fullness, which means you may eat less overall.

Supporting Long-Term Balance

Removing carbs and sugar from your diet doesn't just disrupt the immediate cycle of blood sugar swings; it also supports long-term metabolic health. By reducing insulin spikes and fostering blood sugar stability, these diets can help lower the risk of insulin resistance and related conditions like type 2 diabetes.

It's worth noting that while cutting out carbs and sugar can offer many benefits, the diet should still emphasize nutrient-dense foods like non-starchy vegetables, quality proteins, and healthy fats to ensure a balanced intake of vitamins and minerals.

By breaking the cycle of blood sugar highs and lows, a no-carb or no-sugar diet provides a foundation for steady energy, improved appetite control, and better overall metabolic health.

The Health Risks of High-Carb and High-Sugar Consumption

Eating too many high-carb and high-sugar foods can have serious health consequences. Science has consistently established a link between diets with large amounts of carbohydrates and sugars and an increased risk for certain life-threatening diseases.

The first risk is *diabetes*. High-carb foods often lead to sharp spikes in blood sugar levels, which if left unchecked can eventually cause type-2 diabetes. This disease causes considerable damage to the body's organs, including the heart and kidneys, while also significantly increasing the risk of other life-threatening ailments such as heart disease, stroke, and hypertension.

Heart disease is another consequence of consuming too many sugary treats or processed foods. Eating "empty" calories from these sources contributes to weight gain over time and increases the number of fat deposits in one's bloodstream. This fat buildup slowly clogs up arteries, leading to serious heart complications such as an enlarged heart, chest pain, or even a deadly cardiac arrest.

Obesity is closely linked to both diabetes and heart disease, as well as a host of other ailments such as joint pain, sleep apnea, and mental disorders such as depression or anxiety. Excess consumption of refined carbs leads to higher calorie intake than what our bodies need to burn off; when this excess energy cannot be used efficiently it begins to accumulate in our bodies resulting in weight gain over time.

Hypertension is yet another health risk associated with excessive carb consumption due to its tendency to raise one's blood pressure levels significantly. Sugary drinks that contain fructose are known to increase LDL cholesterol while simultaneously causing salt retention–two major contributors towards the development of high blood pressure; eating sugary snacks like cakes or pastries may also contribute indirectly by raising triglyceride levels in the bloodstream that help regulate hypertension but can be thrown out of balance by ingesting excess simple carbs like those found in desserts or sweet treats.

Stroke can be caused more directly by poorly regulated diabetes or hypertension–two conditions heavily linked with consuming an abundance of processed food that contain large amounts of starch or sugar molecules (glucose). Excessive consumption of these substances has been proven multiple times through studies performed on human subjects; they are known to increase the risk of stroke when not managed properly due to their tendency to raise both blood sugar levels as well as blood pressure significantly over time without proper care & attention being paid towards them respectively.

Finally, artificial sweeteners used widely throughout many products labeled as 'low fat' or 'diet' can also cause negative side effects in some individuals who may react adversely towards certain chemicals contained within them; headaches, nausea, dizziness along with digestive issues are among reported cases related to turning towards artificially sweetened products instead of natural ones like honey or maple syrup which still offer caloric benefits but far fewer possible health risks compared with their artificially produced counterparts.

It is important for individuals looking for better nutrition options to realize that managing carbohydrate intake along with reducing processed food consumption can play a huge role in improving overall well-being & keeping ailments associated with high-carb/high-sugar diets at bay altogether. Moderate intakes rather than extreme abstinence from either macronutrient group should always be encouraged; doing so will ensure good health & reduce your chances of developing serious diseases considerably over time!

The Benefits of a No-Carb/No-Sugar Diet

A no-carb, no-sugar diet has some potential benefits including:

1. *Weight Loss*: Cutting out both carbs and sugar can lead to an overall reduction in caloric intake, leading to weight loss. This is because carbohydrates and sugars are often sources of empty calories that can cause weight gain when consumed in excess.
2. *Reduced Sugar Cravings*: Eliminating sugar from the diet may help reduce cravings since it eliminates easy access to sweet treats throughout the day. By cutting out this source of temptation, one may find it easier to avoid eating sweets altogether.
3. *Improved Mental Clarity*: Reducing sugar intake can lead to more stable blood sugar levels which may result in improved mental clarity and focus since the body won't be constantly fluctuating between high and low energy states due to sudden influxes of refined sugar energy on top of regular carb consumption during meals & snacks.
4. *Reduced Risk of Diabetes & Heart Disease*: Limiting simple carbohydrates like refined sugar can reduce one's risk for developing type-2 diabetes as well as other heart diseases associated with excessive sugar consumption such as hypertension or high cholesterol levels.

5. ***More Nutritious Food Choices***: Limiting both carbs and sugars will likely inspire one to make healthier food choices such as selecting whole grains over processed flours; similarly opting for protein-rich foods instead like lean meat or legumes over bread & cereals filled with added sugars & starches respectively.

A no-carb/no-sugar diet plan can be a safe and effective way to improve overall health and well-being.

The Cons of a No-Carb/No-Sugar Diet

However, just like any other diet plan, there are some potential drawbacks to this approach. The no-carb/no-sugar diet has significant cons and should be approached with caution.

To begin with, the diet can be difficult to stick to; eliminating either group of macronutrients from one's diet can lead to boredom and a lack of variety that makes it hard for people to remain consistent for extended periods. Additionally, it can lead to nutrient deficiencies by severely cutting out a major source of important vitamins and minerals like calcium, vitamin D, B vitamins, and fiber.

Moreover, the no-carb/no-sugar lifestyle can cause digestive problems due to high consumption of processed foods still containing large amounts of starch or sugar molecules (glucose), even when labeled as "low fat" or "diet" have been linked to an increased risk of certain life-threatening diseases such as diabetes and hypertension if not managed properly.

Artificial sweeteners used widely throughout many products can also cause negative side effects in some individuals who may react adversely towards certain chemicals contained within them; headaches, nausea, dizziness along with digestive issues are among reported cases related to turning towards artificially sweetened products instead of natural ones like honey or maple syrup which still offer caloric benefits but far fewer possible health risks compared with their artificially produced counterparts.

Furthermore, such diets can be expensive since they require higher quality food items such as organic produce and wild-caught seafood that do not contain excessive amounts of refined carbs or sugars. Lastly, although people may achieve success in the short term through this type of extreme dietary change, long-term sustainability is questionable due to its limited nutritional value over extended periods; especially since there are potential dangers involved when tying oneself too strictly down this path without specialist advice tailored towards individual needs.

While a no-carb/no-sugar diet might have some benefits when monitored closely by medical professionals over short periods; these should be viewed cautiously by those considering taking on such an extreme dietary change due to its numerous potential drawbacks both physiologically & psychologically!

Common Myths about This Diet

Low-carb or no-carb diets often come with preconceived notions that can overshadow their benefits. While these diets can be effective for many people, misconceptions about what they entail might deter others from giving them a try. Below, we'll address some of the most common myths and clarify the facts to provide a balanced understanding.

Myth 1: You Must Eliminate All Fruits

Many people believe that low-carb or no-carb diets mean cutting out fruits entirely, but this is a misconception. While fruits do contain natural sugars, not all fruits are created equal in terms of their carbohydrate content.

High-sugar fruits like bananas and grapes are higher in quick-digesting carbs, which can lead to blood sugar spikes if consumed in large amounts. However, lower-carb fruits like berries, such as raspberries, strawberries, and blackberries, are excellent options within a low-carb framework. They are rich in fiber, which helps slow down digestion, and they provide essential vitamins and antioxidants.

Rather than avoiding all fruits, this diet encourages focusing on options that align with your blood sugar and carb intake goals.

Myth 2: This Is Just Another Fad Diet

It's easy to dismiss low-carb eating as a short-lived trend, but its foundation is tied to decades of research and even historical eating habits. For instance, scientific studies have consistently shown that low-carb diets can support weight loss, improve blood sugar control, and lower risk factors for certain chronic diseases.

Additionally, this approach mirrors aspects of ancestral diets, where carbohydrate intake was naturally lower and people relied more on protein and natural fats for sustained energy. These diets weren't "fads"; they were a way of life for survival.

Unlike fleeting diet trends, the low-carb or no-carb approach is supported by evidence and offers sustainable options for those who find it aligns with their health goals.

Myth 3: You'll Always Feel Weak or Tired

A common concern is that cutting carbs will leave you drained of energy. While it's true that some people experience an initial adjustment period, often called the "carb flu," this phase is temporary. During this time, as your body transitions from relying on carbs to burning fat for fuel, you might feel symptoms like fatigue, headaches, or irritability.

However, after this adaptation period, your body enters a state called ketosis, where it efficiently uses fat as its primary energy source. Most people report feeling more consistent energy and mental clarity once they're fat-adapted. It's important to stay hydrated and ensure adequate intake of electrolytes during the transition to help minimize discomfort.

Long-term, low-carb diets do not inherently make you weak or tired—in many cases, they promote sustained energy and reduced blood sugar swings.

Myth 4: You Can't Enjoy Food Anymore

Another myth is that low-carb or no-carb eating eliminates all enjoyment from meals. On the contrary, these diets can open the door to rich, flavorful food experiences. Protein-packed meals and healthy fats like avocados, olive oil, and nuts are not only satisfying but also versatile.

Cooking with spices, herbs, and natural seasonings enhances the flavor of meals, offering dishes that are both delicious and nutritious. From savory steaks with garlic butter to creamy coconut curries or roasted vegetables with olive oil and rosemary, there are countless ways to enjoy food on this diet.

Rather than feeling restricted, many people discover new ingredients and cooking methods that make their meals just as enjoyable, if not more so, than before.

Myth 5: If You Cheat Once, You Ruin Everything

One of the biggest misconceptions about low-carb or no-carb diets is the idea that a single cheat meal undoes all your hard work. While cheat meals can affect the body's transition into ketosis, they don't erase the progress you've made or invalidate your efforts.

Instead of viewing a cheat meal as a failure, it's more productive to see it as a learning moment. For example, what led to the choice? Was it a craving, a social situation, or simply curiosity? This reflection can help you better prepare for similar situations in the future, making you stronger in your dietary habits.

Cheat meals can also help you feel more balanced emotionally. Sometimes allowing yourself a small indulgence prevents feelings of deprivation that could lead to abandoning the diet altogether. Remember, consistency over time is what matters most—not perfection.

The key is to approach cheats with moderation and intention. Jump back into your regular diet immediately after, and the occasional indulgence will have little to no long-term impact on your progress.

Low-carb or no-carb diets often face criticism rooted in misinformation. By understanding the facts behind these myths, it becomes clear that this way of eating isn't about deprivation. Instead, it's about making strategic choices that support your health, offering flexibility, sustainability, and plenty of flavor along the way. Whether it's enjoying fresh berries, tapping into ancestral wisdom, or mastering new recipes, this diet has more to offer than many realize.

Preparing Yourself for the Diet

This restrictive diet could happen successfully only if you take things slow to wean the body off sugar at a pace.

Here are some helpful suggestions to prepare your body for the days ahead.

1. **Take the diet slowly.**

    This is part of the whole diet. Changing your diet gradually is the way to come out successfully from this diet. This diet will be especially harsh for those coming from everyday diet menus full of sugar to none. Going cold turkey will not be good for your mental health as well.

2. **Start limiting or completely removing bread products.**

    This includes items like whole wheat bread, cookies, pastries, bagels, and other baked goods. These products are often high in refined carbohydrates and can contribute to blood sugar spikes, making it harder to maintain balanced energy levels and overall health.

Gradually reducing your intake or swapping them for healthier alternatives, such as whole grains or low-carb options, can make a significant difference.

3. **Eat whole fruits instead of fruit juices.**

   Most fruit juices contain added sugars hiding under nutritional labels in names like fruit juice concentrates, molasses, or high-fructose corn syrup.

4. **Avoid artificial sugars.**

   We are in the process of weaning off sugars. Eating artificial sugars tricks the body into thinking it is ingesting real sugar. This not only defeats the whole purpose of this part of the process but intensifies your sugar cravings. Familiar sugar substitutes include Stevia, Splenda, Equal, Sweet 'N Low, and Nutrasweet.

5. **Start to limit or even cut off the intake of soda, alcohol, and sports drinks.**

   It is a very known fact that sodas are high in sugar. A 12 oz (355ml) can of Coca-Cola has 39g grams of sugar and 20 oz (590 ml). Red Bull Energy Drink in 250ml can have 27g. Sports drinks can often be thought of as healthy drinks since they are marketed to be drinks for athletes or those who exercise. A standard 570 ml of sports drink contains 32g of added sugar.

6. **Also limit drinking chocolate milk, flavored coffees, and iced teas.**

   Start getting used to missing your favorite coffee blend. This one is going to be hard for those who start their days with a coffee in hand but one large order of those coffee cups contains nearly 3 times the amount of sugar in a can of Coke. Iced teas also contain 33g of sugar per 340 ml. If it is possible, you can concoct your tea blend and lessen the sugar you put in the drink. One way to add more flavor to your coffee is by adding a healthy alternative, such as grass-fed butter or Oat milk.

7. **Avoid adding condiments with sugar to food.**

   Namely ketchup, barbecue sauce, teriyaki sauce, and salad dressings.

8. **Replace sugar in recipes with spices such as cinnamon, vanilla, almond, or ginger.**
9. **Reduce intake of favorite sweet snacks and beg off on desserts.**

   No more pastries like muffins, baked goods like cake, or frozen treats like ice cream.

10. **Say no to cereal bars.**

   They seem like healthy bars but they are just like candy bars in terms of sugar content. If you take a look at the ingredients for some of these cereal bars, the number of hidden sugars may surprise you. They look appealing and convenient but they are of no help to the diet you are about to start.

11. **Don't forget to speak with your healthcare provider before starting a drastic change in your diet.**

   The guide of a medical professional will help you choose the appropriate food and also remind you of the risk factors involved in the diet.

Learning How to Read Food Labels

As mentioned in previous chapters, added sugars often disguise themselves as ingredients under unfamiliar names. **These are the sweeteners to look out for on food labels:**

- Agave Nectar
- Barley Malt Syrup
- Brown Sugar
- Brown Rice Syrup
- Cane crystals
- Crystalline fructose
- Glucose
- Dextrose
- Maple Syrup
- Fructose
- Fruit juice concentrate
- Invert sugar
- High-fructose corn syrup
- Honey
- Sucrose
- Maltodextrin
- Maltose

- Malt Syrup
- Corn sweetener
- Molasses
- Palm Sugar
- Raw sugar
- Evaporated Cane Juice
- Cane sugar
- Turbinado Sugar
- Corn Syrup
- Hidden sugars can be found in baked beans and tacos.

Here are some sugar replacements to watch out for. They are often added as ingredients in food products.

- Saccharin
- Aspartame
- Sucralose
- Neotame
- Acesulfame potassium

As you can see, many of these ingredients contain sugar, yet do not have a sugar-sounding name. The easiest way to curb sugar intake is to focus on buying and consuming real, whole foods. Foods contained in some packaging typically have hidden sugars.

As shown, shopping at the grocery store can be challenging when trying to avoid hidden sugars. Many processed and packaged foods, from breakfast cereals to condiments, often contain sneaky sweeteners that can derail efforts to maintain a healthy diet.

To make informed choices, always read ingredient labels carefully, and focus on purchasing fresh produce, lean proteins, and whole grains. Sticking to the outer aisles of the grocery store, where fresh and unprocessed items are typically kept, can also help you avoid added sugars.

Want to learn more tips and tricks for navigating the grocery store like a pro?

Focusing on the Right Foods

Always aim to eat at least three times a day even as you follow the no-carb, no-sugar diet. The standard day starts with a healthy breakfast, followed by lunch and dinner without any intake of carbohydrates and sugar.

Here's a list of what you should include in your diet:

- Eggs
- Non-starchy vegetables
- Nuts and sugar-free nut butter
- Meat and poultry such as chicken, beef, pork, and turkey
- Seafood
- More spices and seasonings
- Olive oi
- Berries: Blueberries, blackberries, and strawberries
- Unsweetened teas
- Avocado

Focus on lean meats and seafood in the main courses to provide you with energy to power through the day. Fish like salmon, trout, tuna, and wild-caught fish are great choices for main course meals. These help you feel and stay full, thus reducing sugar cravings throughout your day.

Suggested Menu

Day 1

Breakfast: Oatmeal or cooked eggs (preferably egg whites only)

Lunch: Grilled meat (chicken or seafood) with salad

Dinner: Tuna salad

Day 2

Breakfast: Bacon and eggs

Lunch: Grilled or fried fish with some olive oil

Dinner: Shrimp pasta with vegetables

Day 3

Breakfast: No-carb bread

Lunch: Chicken breasts and garlic spinach

Dinner: Glazed chicken thighs

Day 4

Breakfast: Roasted veggies

Lunch: Grilled lamb

Dinner: Salmon with vegetables

Day 5

Breakfast: Avocado and smoked salmon on a slice of no-carb bread

Lunch: Grilled turkey breast with a side of roasted Brussels sprouts and a sprinkle of almonds

Dinner: Zucchini noodles with garlic shrimp, tossed in a light olive oil and lemon sauce

Day 6

Breakfast: Vegetable noodles

Lunch: Smoothies, zero-carb pizza

Dinner: Grilled chicken wings

Day 7

Breakfast: Scrambled eggs with sausage, unsweetened yogurt

Lunch: Broccoli and Tomato salad with nuts

Dinner: Grilled salmon

Day 8

Breakfast: Chia seed oatmeal with cantaloupes

Lunch: Tofu soup with mushrooms and lots of seasonings

Dinner: Salad bowl of tomatoes, carrots, celery sticks, peppers, lettuce

Day 9

Breakfast: Poached eggs with slices of ham

Lunch: Grilled steak and asparagus

Dinner: Lettuce wraps, salmon, cucumber, and tuna salad

Day 10

Breakfast: Boiled eggs and No-carb banana cake bread

Lunch: Lettuce-wrapped burgers

Dinner: Protein smoothie

A diet with no carbohydrates means the dieters will rely on other food sources for their food intake. You could consider having high-protein meals during the diet to not lose muscle mass.

This is helpful for bodybuilders or other athletes who wish to increase muscle mass while still on a no-carb, no-sugar diet. Most bacon strips have sugar added to them for additional flavor. Be conscious to choose the options with the "No Sugar

Added" label. Go to the butcher as much as you possibly can to be able to get the right cut of pork belly strips. Stay away from brands that have even 2g of sugar on their labels.

It is okay to eat eggs even on a no-carb diet. Hard-boiled eggs are great as breakfast and snack options. They can also be added to vegetable salads. They can be cooked as an omelet and paired with bacon.

Peanut oil and safflower oil have 0 carbohydrates. These oils apart from canola oil can help in adding flavor to food. Grilled meat with a lot of spices and brushed with oils make for a good stand-alone dinner and make cravings for sides like mashed potatoes or sweet corn easier.

When eating out, always order plain water instead of the usual fruit juice or soda. Get extra vegetables if available. When shopping, avoid the chips and candies section at all costs. Stock your fridge with meat, grass-fed butter, coconut oil, olive oil, eggs, fish, and herbs. Unsweetened yogurt can be eaten as a dessert. It is a good alternative to ice cream and other sweets.

Snacks in between could be nuts or cauliflowers and mushrooms that will keep your cravings at bay and make you feel full. It is important to listen to your body or drink herbal teas when tempted to cave.

Low-carb oatmeal substitutes for breakfast or snacks

1. **Chia Seed Oatmeal**

   Chia seeds are great sources of vitamins and minerals such as potassium, magnesium, and calcium. They are also high in omega-3 fatty acids and fiber. They resemble the texture of oats and they are prepared just the same. They only require water since they expand when soaked up. Just like oats, they are perfect with fruits for breakfast.

2. **Flaxseed Oatmeal**

   Flaxseed helps in improving digestion and contributes to weight loss. They help lower cholesterol and blood sugar levels. Flaxseed has zero grams of net carbs, which is perfect for this diet.

3. **Hemp Heart Seeds Oatmeal**

   Hemp heart seeds are seeds of the hemp plant. They are high in nutritional value and help with muscle growth. They are excellent macronutrients and just as easy to prepare.

Snack ideas

1. **Homemade trail mix**
   - Mix unsweetened coconut flakes, pecans, and pumpkin seeds.
   - Tuna salad lettuce wraps
2. **Stuffed avocado**
   - Fill the avocado with tuna, salmon, or shrimp. Then top with scrambled eggs.
3. **Carrot sticks with minced garlic in olive oil.**
   - You can also use Hummus as a dip. Make sure that there is no sugar.
4. **Strawberry smoothie**
   - Blend unsweetened milk, fresh strawberries, chia seeds, and vanilla extract.
5. **No carb guacamole**
   - Mash avocados and add onion, garlic, lime juice, and a bit of salt in a bowl.
6. **Kale chips**
   - Bake bite-sized kale pieces with olive oil, garlic, and salt.
7. **Toasted pumpkin seeds in cinnamon**
   - Combine toasted seeds and cinnamon. Spread seeds on a baking sheet and bake until golden brown.

8. **Unsweetened yogurt with nuts**
    - Always keep in mind to look for the unsweetened variety. Add a handful of nuts and sprinkle with cinnamon.
9. **Egg salad with avocado**
    - Mash avocado with hard-boiled eggs. Sprinkle a bit of salt and pepper. Best to eat with lettuce wraps.

Food to Stay Away From

Curbing sugar cravings can be pretty hard when starting. Sweet lozenges may help with sugar cravings. Also, look for herbs or tonics that can block sugar taste receptors on the tongue to suppress sweet taste.

To start, here's a list of what you should start removing from your diet:

- Grains: wheat, corn, and rice
- Beans: kidney, black, and pinto
- Legumes: Lentils and chickpeas
- Starchy vegetables such as potatoes, sweet potatoes, beets, parsnips, winter squash
- Candies
- Condiments like ketchup, salad dressings, barbecue sauce, teriyaki sauce
- Sweeteners
- Alcohol
- Soda
- Dairy

- Baked goods such as bread, crackers, cookies, and cakes
- Most fruits (berries are typically better than others)

As mentioned in the preparation process, cereal bars are often marketed as healthy breakfast substitutes but these are high in added sugar content. Breakfast is considered the most important meal of the day. Start your day with high-protein foods like egg whites instead of cereals.

Also, avoid packaged snacks. Most of the snacks contain flour and sugar. Reach for nuts instead when you crave sweet snacks. There are almonds, hazelnuts, walnuts, and peanuts. If available, go for cashews, pecans, pistachios, or macadamia nuts. These all have to be in a serving smaller than one hand since they still contain small amounts of carbohydrates.

Although fruits are generally healthy, for this diet there are a lot of fruits you should look out for in terms of sugar content and carbohydrates. Apples, bananas, plantains, and dates should be avoided. Do not buy oranges, passion fruits, pomegranates, grapes, figs, pears, and mangoes at the fruit section of the grocery. Also avoid kiwi, kumquat, and lychee. Aim for berries, such as blueberries as they are high in antioxidants.

Foods to Eat More

1. **Vegetables**

   If you miss the taste of bread, shredded zucchini, or yellow squash, make a great alternative. For mashed potatoes, mashed cauliflowers can be made as substitutes.

   Munch on carrots for snacks. Always have a bowl of broccoli ready in your fridge when you are tempted to reach for chocolate bars. Have a lot of asparagus as a side meal.

2. **Herbs**

   Add herbs to water like mint, cilantro, rosemary, or sage. If added together in huge amounts and then soaked overnight, they can make a bottle drink alternative to sodas.

3. **Protein-style versions**

   There are burger or sandwich options that you can beg off on buns. This is a good way to enjoy a burger meal without carbs. Instead of the usual bread buns, ask for vegetable alternatives like lettuce or other greens. Also, request an order without condiments.

4. **Water**

   Water is your best friend in a no-carb, no-sugar diet. It is always the best advice to not forget to drink water particularly when you are on a restrictive diet. In times when you crave the taste of sodas or iced teas, putting in lemon or cucumber slices in iced cold water will do the trick.

5. **Variety of Spices**

   No sugar does not also mean no spice. If you remove the flavor of food from the diet, it will make the diet unsustainable. Look into spices or seasonings to add excitement to your meals. If you wish to have coffee, have black coffee topped with cinnamon. Sprinkle cardamom with unsweetened yogurt.

Here are some common mistakes that a dieter needs to be wary of while on this diet:

1. *Too much protein*

   Since carbohydrates are being restricted, some people tend to overindulge in proteins. They can help in making you feel full and stave off the carb-hunger but if your goal is losing weight in the process, it is very important to watch your protein intake as well.

2. *Not eating fat*

Eliminating carbohydrates and sugar in your usual diet means your body is likely to look for whatever filling substitute is available. Do not be afraid to reach out to fats to compensate for the loss of carbs in the diet.

Note that you should stick with healthy fats. (Yes, fats can be healthy!) Stay with foods like avocado and wild-caught salmon. Choosing fatty cuts of meat in moderation is good to stave off hunger. Since the diet is already very restrictive, you must find ways to sustain yourself and not get sick in the process. Your body needs enough energy to function and also to get nutrition.

3. *Not getting enough sodium*

In a no-carb, no-sugar diet, the insulin levels of your body go down as well as sodium. Low sodium levels can become problematic for your kidneys. This is why some feel lightheaded and fatigued in this type of diet. Add a little bit more salt to your food or drink meat broth every day.

4. *Not getting enough vitamin C*

Vitamin C boosts the function of the immune system. It contributes to the immune defense by supporting the cellular functions of both the innate and adaptive immune systems. It is also a potent antioxidant. Vitamin C supplements prevent and treat respiratory and systemic functions.

When we think of a fruit rich in vitamin C, we immediately think of the orange. But the orange, however natural, is not low in sugar. There are other sources of vitamin C that we should eat and still maintain the no-sugar diet. Zucchini boasts 58 mg of Vitamin C. They are best consumed unpeeled as the outer part is the most nutrient-dense portion.

Red and green bell peppers also contain 152 mg of Vitamin C.

Kale, broccoli, Brussels sprouts, and cauliflower are also excellent sources of Vitamin C.

5. *Missing out on fruits*

Although a lot of familiar fruits have significant amounts of carbohydrates and sugar, there are fruits we can indulge in without feeling guilty. Berries are very versatile.

They can be added to yogurts for breakfast or snacks. Strawberries, blackberries, and raspberries are low in sugar and high in fiber. Melons or cantaloupes are very refreshing.

They are low in carbohydrates and also good sources of vitamins A and C. They are high in water content which is great against electrolyte imbalance while in the diet. Stone fruits like cherries, peaches, plums, nectarines, and apricots are low in carbohydrates and high in dietary fiber. Papaya and peach are great choices too.

6. *Throwing in the towel too early*

This is why preparation is as important as the whole process. The preparation stage helps your body adjust to the diet more easily. Carbs and sugar seem unavoidable and your body has already gotten used to ingesting them every single day.

Feelings of uneasiness in the first few days are normal. Even with all the preparation, your mind may take time to adjust. It is very important to be patient to come out successfully and see evidence that results in weight loss and sugar levels even just after two weeks.

Reminders:

1. It can be very difficult to find foods with no carbs and sugar on grocery shelves. Write out a list of things to buy along with their alternatives before going shopping.
2. Do not skip meals as these will make you feel lightheaded in the process and may cause you to

overeat on your next meal and crave more of the banned food sources.
3. Forgive yourself for slip-ups and celebrate your successes.
4. Always read the labels. Double-check before going to the counter since you might miss the added sugar content in unfamiliar names.
5. Aim for sustainable weight loss to make you feel your best after the weeks of dieting.

Understanding Sugar Cravings: What Your Body Is Really Telling You

Sugar cravings can feel overwhelming and uncontrollable, leaving many people wondering why their bodies are begging for something sweet. At the heart of these cravings lies a fascinating interplay of biological processes and nutritional imbalances. Understanding the root causes can help you manage your cravings and support your overall health.

Biological Reasons You Crave Sugar

Imbalanced Blood Sugar Levels

One of the most common reasons behind sugar cravings is an imbalance in blood sugar levels. When your blood sugar drops too low, your body signals a need for quick energy, often in the form of sugary or carbohydrate-rich foods.

Here's how it works:

- *After a sugar spike* - Eating sugary or refined-carb foods can cause your blood sugar to rise rapidly. This triggers a surge of insulin to bring blood sugar levels back down. Sometimes, insulin works too efficiently, leading to a sharp blood sugar drop or "sugar crash."

- *During a sugar crash* - The sudden drop leaves you feeling tired, shaky, or irritable, and your brain sends out cravings for sugar to quickly replenish energy stores.

If you find yourself in a cycle of sugar highs and lows, focusing on balanced meals with protein, healthy fats, and fiber can help stabilize your blood sugar and reduce cravings.

Gut Microbiome Signals

Your gut microbiome plays a surprisingly large role in your cravings. The trillions of bacteria in your gut communicate with your brain, influencing not just digestion but also your food preferences. Some bacteria thrive on sugars, and when their numbers grow, they can send signals to encourage you to eat more sugar.

For example, an overgrowth of certain yeast strains, like Candida albicans, may lead to intense sugar cravings. This happens because these microorganisms use sugar as their primary fuel, and craving sugary foods helps them survive and multiply.

Supporting a healthy gut microbiome is key to addressing these types of cravings. Eating a diet rich in prebiotics (found in fiber-rich foods like vegetables) and probiotics (found in fermented foods like yogurt, kimchi, and sauerkraut) can help maintain a balanced gut environment.

Nutrient Deficiencies (Like Magnesium or Chromium)

Your body's cravings aren't always about pleasure; sometimes they're a cry for specific nutrients it lacks. Nutrient deficiencies, especially in magnesium and chromium, are closely linked to sugar cravings and energy regulation.

- *Magnesium*: This essential mineral supports over 300 metabolic processes in the body, including those responsible for blood sugar regulation. Without enough magnesium, the body struggles to properly use insulin and balance blood sugar levels, leading to cravings for quick energy sources like sugary foods. Foods high in magnesium include spinach, almonds, pumpkin seeds, and dark chocolate (unsweetened or low-sugar varieties).
- *Chromium*: Chromium is a trace mineral that enhances the action of insulin, promoting stable blood sugar levels. A chromium deficiency can impair your body's ability to manage blood sugar, triggering cravings to compensate for the dip in energy. To boost chromium intake, incorporate foods like broccoli, eggs, green beans, and nuts into your diet.

It's worth noting that deficiencies in zinc, B-vitamins, and omega-3 fatty acids may also play a role in sugar cravings, as they impact energy production and brain function. A nutrient-dense, balanced diet can be one of the most effective strategies to address these deficiencies and reduce cravings.

Sugar cravings often stem from blood sugar imbalances, gut health, or nutritional deficiencies. By stabilizing blood sugar, supporting gut health, and meeting nutrient needs, you can reduce cravings and help your body rely on healthier energy sources over time.

Emotional Triggers & Habits

For many people, eating isn't just about hunger; it's deeply tied to emotions and habits. Emotional triggers and routines often influence what, when, and how we eat, sometimes leading to patterns that feel difficult to break.

By understanding these influences, you can start to identify and address the root causes of cravings or overeating. Below, we'll take a closer look at how emotions and habits shape your relationship with food.

Eating for Comfort, Reward, or Stress

Food has long been associated with emotions. For some, eating becomes a way to deal with feelings like stress, sadness, or even joy. This is often referred to as emotional eating. Here's how it works:

- ***Comfort Eating*** - Stress, loneliness, or sadness can lead you to crave foods associated with comfort, often items high in sugar, fat, or carbohydrates. These "feel-good" foods can temporarily activate the brain's reward system by releasing dopamine, a chemical linked to pleasure. However, the relief is short-lived, often followed by guilt or regret.
- ***Using Food as a Reward*** - Some people tie eating to accomplishments or treat food as a reward for surviving a stressful day. For example, you might think, "I had a hard day; I deserve this dessert." While this may soothe you in the moment, it can create a habit of linking achievement or relief to food, reinforcing an emotional dependency.
- ***Stress-Based Eating*** - Chronic stress leads to the release of cortisol, a hormone that increases appetite and can trigger cravings for sugary or fatty foods. This is because your body perceives stress as a need for extra energy, and sugary foods provide quick fuel. Over time, this cycle can become automatic, leading you to use food as a coping mechanism even when you're not physically hungry.

Association with Routines

Habits and routines also play a significant role in shaping your eating behaviors, often without you even realizing it.

- ***Evening Sugar Cravings*** - For many, sugar becomes part of a routine, such as having dessert after dinner. Over time, your brain learns to anticipate that sugary reward after a meal, and the craving becomes automatic—even if your body doesn't physically need it.
- ***Food Pairing Habits*** - Some cravings develop from associating certain foods with specific activities or settings. For instance, you might always crave popcorn at the movies or a slice of cake at a celebration. While these aren't inherently bad, the repeated pairing of specific foods with certain situations can create a habitual craving every time you encounter that scenario.

Breaking the Cycle

Addressing emotional triggers and habits takes self-awareness and focused effort. Here are some strategies to help untangle these patterns and build a healthier relationship with food:

1. ***Pause and Reflect***: When you feel the urge to eat, ask yourself if you're truly hungry or if the craving is tied to an emotional state. This pause allows you to identify the underlying reason for your desire to eat.
2. ***Find Alternative Coping Mechanisms***: If you're eating for emotional reasons, try other activities that can provide comfort or release stress. A walk,

journaling, deep breathing, or talking to a friend can be helpful substitutes for turning to food.
3. ***Rewire Associations***: To break habitual cravings, change up your routines. For example, if you associate dinner with dessert, replace dessert with an herbal tea or a short walk. Over time, your brain will adapt to the new pattern.
4. ***Add Mindful Eating Practices***: Pay close attention to what you eat, savoring each bite without distractions. This technique can help you tune into your body's true hunger and fullness cues, while also reducing the influence of emotional triggers.
5. ***Plan Ahead***: If you tend to eat under stress, prepare healthier options ahead of time that satisfy cravings without derailing your goals. Having nutritious snacks on hand can help you make better choices when emotions run high.

Food is deeply connected to our emotions and habits, so it's natural to find yourself reaching for comfort foods or indulging in routines out of habit. But by identifying emotional triggers and reassessing automatic behaviors, you can create a healthier, more intentional relationship with food. Building self-awareness and gradually implementing small changes will help you shift from reactive eating to mindful, balanced choices that truly nourish your body and mind.

What to Do Instead of Giving In to Sugar Cravings

Sugar cravings can feel overwhelming, but the good news is that they are often short-lived. If you can manage those moments in a constructive way, you'll find that cravings pass and you feel more in control of your choices. Below, we'll explore some effective strategies to help you manage sugar cravings without derailing your goals.

1. **Use the 3-Minute Delay Rule**

    Have you heard the saying, "Pause before you act"? That's the philosophy behind the 3-minute delay rule. When a craving hits, tell yourself to wait three minutes before giving in. Why does this work? Often, cravings are fleeting and lose their intensity after just a few moments. By delaying your reaction, you create space to make a more mindful decision.

    During those three minutes, focus on something else. Here are a few quick options to help you reset:

    - ***Drink a glass of water***: Hydration can diminish cravings because thirst is often confused with hunger or a need for sugar.
    - ***Take deep breaths***: Cravings can be amplified by stress, so slowing your breath can calm both your body and mind.

- *Move your body*: A little light activity, like stretching your arms or walking around your space, can distract you and reduce your focus on the craving.

After three minutes, your craving may feel less urgent. At that point, you can more easily assess whether eating something (and choosing a healthier option) aligns with your goals. It's like hitting a mental reset button that allows you to regain control.

2. **Distract Yourself with an Activity**

Cravings thrive on attention. The more you obsess over that piece of cake or candy bar, the harder it becomes to resist. Shifting your focus to an engaging activity is a powerful way to redirect your thoughts and weaken the craving.

<u>Here are a few replacement activities to try:</u>

- *Get moving*: A quick walk, some light exercise, or a short yoga session can work wonders. Physical activity not only distracts you but also releases endorphins, which improve your mood and help reduce stress-induced cravings.
- *Reach out to a friend*: Call, text, or even FaceTime someone. Engaging in conversation keeps your brain busy and shifts the attention away from food.

- ***Chew sugar-free gum or mints***: This gives you a sweet sensation without the actual sugar. Plus, it occupies your mouth, making it less tempting to snack.
- ***Dive into a hobby***: Whether it's sketching, knitting, gardening, or playing an instrument, hobbies are great for keeping your hands and mind busy. Activities like these help distract you from cravings while also boosting your sense of accomplishment.

By breaking the cycle of focusing on sugar, you'll likely notice that the craving diminishes over time.

3. **Opt for Healthier Alternatives**

Sometimes the craving for food is too persistent to ignore entirely, and that's okay. Instead of trying to power through without eating anything, opt for a healthier substitution that satisfies your taste buds without spiking your blood sugar.

Here are some nutritious replacement options:

- ***Fresh berries***: Strawberries, blueberries, or raspberries offer natural sweetness along with fiber, vitamins, and antioxidants to balance their small sugar content.
- ***A handful of nuts or seeds***: Almonds, walnuts, or sunflower seeds provide healthy fats and

protein, which can help stabilize blood sugar and keep you feeling full longer.

- *A spoonful of nut butter*: A small amount of almond or peanut butter (without added sugar) can offer a creamy, satisfying treat.
- *Greek yogurt with cinnamon*: Unsweetened yogurt delivers protein, while cinnamon provides a hint of natural sweetness and added health benefits.

By keeping these alternatives on hand, you can meet your cravings halfway without compromising your goals.

4. **Hydrate with Electrolyte Water or Herbal Tea'**

Cravings can often be a sign that your body is in need of something other than sugar, like hydration or essential nutrients. Drinking the right liquids can be a powerful tool to curb cravings.

- *Electrolyte Water*: Sometimes your body mistakes thirst or low electrolyte levels for hunger. Electrolyte water restores essential minerals like potassium and sodium, which are necessary for energy regulation and hydration. You can find unsweetened electrolyte drinks or make your own by adding a pinch of salt and a squeeze of fresh lemon or lime to plain water.

- *Herbal Tea*: Warm and soothing, herbal teas come in an array of natural flavors that can help satisfy your sweet tooth. For example, cinnamon tea has a naturally sweet aroma, mint tea feels refreshing, and chamomile tea can help calm your nerves if you're feeling stressed. Sipping tea also provides a comforting ritual, creating a pause that can help dissipate the craving.

Drinking enough water and other healthy liquids throughout the day can also help reduce the frequency of cravings, as your body becomes less likely to confuse thirst with hunger.

5. Build Long-Term Habits for Success

Managing sugar cravings isn't just about saying no in the moment. It's about setting yourself up for long-term success by developing habits that reduce the intensity and frequency of cravings over time.

Here are some tips to support sustainable change:

- *Balance your meals*: Include protein, healthy fats, and fiber in each meal to keep your blood sugar stable and prevent sudden spikes and crashes.

- ***Get enough sleep***: Poor sleep disrupts hormones that regulate hunger and satiety, which can make cravings harder to resist.
- ***Reduce stress***: High stress can trigger emotional eating. Practice stress-reducing techniques like meditation, deep breathing, or engaging in relaxing activities.
- ***Keep temptation out of sight***: If sugary treats are within easy reach, you're more likely to give in. Stock your pantry with healthier snacks instead.
- ***Practice mindfulness***: Stay present while eating and really savor your food. This helps you build a stronger connection to your body's actual needs, reducing the urge to eat out of boredom or habit.

Sugar cravings don't have to control you. By applying simple yet effective strategies like pausing before acting, distracting yourself, choosing healthier alternatives, and ensuring hydration, you can take charge of your cravings. Over time, these practices will become second nature, and you'll feel more confident and empowered in your ability to make choices that align with your health goals. Remember, cravings are temporary, but the benefits of resisting them can be long-lasting!

Herbal or Supplement Support for Cravings

Sometimes, sugar cravings can feel tough to manage, and you might wonder if there are natural remedies or supplements that can help. While these options aren't magic fixes, some herbs and supplements may play a role in reducing cravings. Remember, it's essential to check with your doctor before trying any of these to ensure they're safe for you.

1. **Gymnema Sylvestre**

   Gymnema Sylvestre is a plant known for its ability to reduce the taste of sweetness. When taken as a tea or supplement, it may help curb sugar cravings by dulling your sweet taste receptors. This means sugary treats may not taste as appealing after consuming Gymnema. Plus, some research suggests it might support healthy blood sugar levels, which can also help manage cravings.

2. **Cinnamon**

   Cinnamon is a common kitchen spice that might do more than flavor your food. It's believed to help stabilize blood sugar levels, preventing those sharp spikes and crashes that often lead to sugar cravings. Adding a bit of cinnamon to your meals, smoothies, or herbal tea could help you feel satisfied for longer. You can also find cinnamon supplements, but make sure to speak to your doctor before using them regularly.

3. **L-Glutamine**

   L-Glutamine is an amino acid that your body uses for various functions, including managing energy. Some experts suggest that it can help reduce sugar cravings by feeding your brain with an alternative energy source. If you find yourself craving sugar throughout the day, taking L-glutamine as a supplement—or even mixing it into water as a powder—may help. But, as with any supplement, it's best to consult your healthcare provider before use.

   While these herbs and supplements may support your efforts to manage sugar cravings, they're not a substitute for a balanced diet and healthy habits. It's also crucial to work with your physician or a healthcare professional before adding anything new to your routine. They can help you determine the right dose and ensure that these remedies are safe and fit well with any other medications or health conditions you have.

   Herbs like Gymnema Sylvestre and cinnamon, along with the supplement L-glutamine, might offer some extra help in managing sugar cravings. When used alongside mindful eating, hydration, and emotional awareness, they can become part of your toolkit for reducing cravings and building healthier habits.

Curated Recipes

Added to this guide are various recipes to choose from. Feel free to draw inspiration from this list, and make your variations!

Grilled Lamb

Ingredients:

- 1-1/2 lb. baby spinach leaves
- 3 tbsp. dried oregano, chopped
- 1/4 cup lemon juice
- 1/4 cup olive oil
- 2 tbsp. ground cumin
- 1 tsp. crushed red pepper
- 1 tbsp. coarse sea salt
- 1 tbsp. squeezed juice from an orange
- 3 cloves garlic
- 2 yellow onions, chopped
- cooking spray

Instructions:

1. In a 2-gallon zip bag, put the lamb together with the lemon juice, oregano, cumin, and salt.
2. Close the bag and refrigerate overnight
3. Puree onions, garlic, some orange juice, and olive oil in a blender.
4. Transfer to a small bowl with a cover.
5. Chill overnight.
6. Mix sea salt, red pepper, and cumin in a small bowl
7. Remove refrigerated lamb and let it sit for 30 minutes.
8. Preheat the grill to medium.

9. Place lamb on the grill and coat with some cooking spray or oil.
10. Grill lamb for one and a half hours over medium heat.
11. Remove the lamb from the grill.
12. Serve hot.

Avocado and Smoked Salmon on a Slice of No-Carb Bread

Ingredients:

- 1 ripe avocado
- 2 slices of no-carb bread
- 4 oz. smoked salmon, sliced
- Fresh lemon juice
- Salt and pepper to taste

Instructions:

1. Begin by slicing the avocado in half and removing the pit.
2. Scoop out the flesh into a small bowl and mash it with a fork.
3. Add a squeeze of fresh lemon juice and salt and pepper to taste.
4. Toast two slices of no-carb bread until lightly golden.
5. Spread the mashed avocado mixture onto the toast.
6. Arrange slices of smoked salmon on top of the avocado spread.
7. Drizzle a little more lemon juice on top and sprinkle with additional salt and pepper if desired.
8. Serve immediately and enjoy your delicious, low-carb avocado toast with smoked salmon.

Roasted Veggies

Ingredients:

- 1/2 lb. turnips
- 1/2 lb. carrots
- 1/2 lb. parsnips
- 2 shallots, peeled
- 1/4 tsp. ground black pepper
- 1 tbsp. extra-virgin olive oil
- 6 cloves garlic
- 3/4 tsp. kosher salt
- 2 tbsp. fresh rosemary needles

Instructions:

1. First, cut vegetables into bite-sized pieces.
2. Set the oven to 400°F.
3. Mix all the ingredients in a baking dish.
4. Roast the vegetables for 25 minutes until brown and tender.
5. Toss and roast again for 20–25 minutes.
6. Serve and enjoy while hot.

Ground Beef Stroganoff

Ingredients:

- 1 lb. 80% lean ground beef
- 2 tbsp. butter
- 1 clove garlic, minced
- 10 oz. sliced mushrooms
- 1 tbsp. fresh parsley, chopped
- 1 tbsp. fresh lemon juice
- salt
- pepper
- 2 tbsp. water

Instructions:

1. Heat the large skillet over medium heat.
2. Put in the butter, letting it melt.
3. Add in the garlic and wait until it turns brown
4. Add beef and season with salt and pepper.
5. When the garlic turns brown, add the beef. Season with salt and pepper.
6. Drain some of the oil from the skillet.
7. Add the mushroom to the leftover oil and cook for 2 minutes. Add water.
8. Reduce the heat to low. Add the lemon juice.
9. Garnish with parsley and serve immediately.

Banana Bread

Ingredients:

- 1 cup olive oil mayonnaise
- 2 eggs
- 4 medium ripe bananas, mashed
- 2 tsp. vanilla extract
- 2 cups unbleached all-purpose flour
- 1 cup whole wheat flour
- 3/4 cup Brown Xylitol
- 2 tsp. baking soda
- 2 tsp. sea salt
- 2 tsp. cinnamon
- 1 tsp. baking powder
- Optional: flax, nuts, wheat germ, or whey protein

Instructions:

1. Preheat the oven to 350°F.
2. In a large mixing bowl, mix in banana, mayonnaise, eggs, and vanilla extract.
3. Combine the remaining dry ingredients in a different container.
4. Combine both mixtures by adding the dry one to the wet mixture.
5. Stir in the optional ingredients if desired.

6. Place the batter into a couple of loaf pans. Make sure to grease the pans first.
7. Place in the oven for about 45 to 50 minutes.
8. Let stand for 10 minutes. Remove from pan to finish cooling.
9. Serve and enjoy.

Chicken breasts and Garlic Spinach

Ingredients:

- 4 chicken breasts
- 2 tbsp olive oil
- Salt and pepper to taste
- 1 tsp dried oregano
- 1 tsp dried basil
- 1 tsp garlic powder
- 4 cloves of garlic, minced
- 6 cups of fresh spinach leaves

Instructions:

1. Preheat oven to 375°F (190°C).
2. Season both sides of the chicken breasts with salt, pepper, dried oregano, dried basil, and garlic powder.
3. Heat olive oil in a large skillet over medium-high heat.
4. Add minced garlic to the skillet and cook for 1-2 minutes until fragrant.
5. Place seasoned chicken breasts into the skillet and cook for 5 minutes on each side until golden brown.
6. Transfer the chicken breasts to a baking dish and bake in the preheated oven for 20-25 minutes or until internal temperature reaches 165°F (74°C).

7. While the chicken is cooking, add fresh spinach leaves to the same skillet used to cook the chicken.
8. Sauté the spinach for 2-3 minutes until wilted.
9. Serve the chicken on top of the sautéed spinach and garnish with freshly chopped parsley, if desired.

Healthy Green Smoothie

Ingredients:

- 1 cup fresh spinach
- 1/2 tsp. mint extract or to taste
- Optional: 1/4 tsp. peppermint liquid Stevia

Instructions:

1. Gather the ingredients.
2. Add them to a high-powered blender.
3. Turn on the blender.
4. Add them to the glass and freeze for 5 minutes.
5. Serve and enjoy.

Red Velvet Molten Lava Cake

Ingredients:

- 2 tbsp. coconut flour
- 1 tbsp. unsweetened cocoa powder
- 1 tbsp. ground flaxseed meal
- 1/2 tsp. baking powder
- 1/4 tsp. salt
- 1/4 cup 1% milk
- 1/4 tsp. vanilla extract
- 2 eggs
- 1 tsp. chocolate liquid stevia, or 1/2 cup of sugar-free sweetener
- 85% dark chocolate bars, broken into pieces
- 3 drops of red food coloring

Instructions:

1. Mix the coconut flour, cocoa powder, flaxseed, baking powder, and salt.
2. In a separate bowl, whisk the milk, eggs, vanilla extract, stevia, and food coloring together.
3. Pour the dry mixture into the wet mixture. Stir until combined.
4. Adjust food coloring to the redness you desire.
5. Spray oil on a couple of microwave-safe mugs or ramekins.

6. Pour batter into each container.
7. Insert chocolate pieces in the center of each batter.
8. Microwave one cake at a time for about one and a half minutes.
9. Serve and enjoy while warm.

Grilled Steak and Asparagus

Ingredients:

- 2 lbs. asparagus
- 4 pcs. ribeye steaks, about 1" thick each
- salt
- pepper
- olive oil

Instructions:

1. Preheat the grill to high heat.
2. Trim the ends of the asparagus and place them in a dish or resealable plastic bag.
3. Season with olive oil, salt, and pepper.
4. Place steak on the grill and cook for about 4 to 5 minutes on each side for medium-rare doneness.
5. Remove from the grill and let rest for 10 minutes before slicing.
6. Place seasoned asparagus on the grill and cook for about 3 to 4 minutes, turning occasionally.
7. Once the asparagus is tender and lightly charred, remove from the grill.
8. Serve grilled asparagus alongside sliced ribeye steaks.

Chicken Masala Crockpot Style

Ingredients:

- 6 boneless skinless chicken breasts, halved lengthwise
- 2 cloves of minced garlic
- 2 tbsp. extra virgin olive oil
- 1 tsp. salt
- 1 tsp. pepper
- 2 cups Marsala wine or chicken broth
- 1 cup of cold water
- 1/2 cup arrowroot powder
- 16 oz. sliced baby Portobello mushrooms
- 3 tbsp. fresh parsley, chopped

Instructions:

1. Grease the slow cooker. Add garlic and oil.
2. Season chicken with salt and pepper on each side and lay in the crockpot.
3. Pour wine over the chicken and cover the crockpot.
4. Cook on high for 3 hours.
5. Mix water with arrowroot and stir until absorbed.
6. Remove chicken from the crockpot and keep warm.
7. Stir in the arrowroot water mixture into the bottom of the crockpot. Add mushrooms.

8. Add back the chicken. Stir well to coat the chicken with sauce and mushrooms.
9. Cover and cook for an additional hour.
10. Serve with a sprinkle of chopped fresh parsley.

Broccoli and Tomato Salad with Nuts and Seeds

Ingredients:

- 2 cups broccoli florets
- 1 cup cherry tomatoes, halved
- ¼ cup chopped almonds
- ¼ cup pumpkin seeds
- 2 tablespoons sunflower seeds
- Salt and pepper to taste

Instructions:

1. In a large bowl, combine the broccoli florets and cherry tomatoes.
2. In a separate pan over medium heat, toast the chopped almonds, pumpkin seeds, and sunflower seeds until slightly golden and fragrant.
3. Add the toasted nuts and seeds to the bowl with the broccoli and tomatoes.
4. Season with salt and pepper, to taste.
5. Toss everything together until well combined.
6. Serve as a side dish or enjoy as a light meal on its own.

Balsamic-Glazed Chicken Thighs

Ingredients:

- 1 tsp. garlic powder
- 1 tsp. dried basil
- 1/2 tsp. salt
- 1/2 tsp. pepper
- 2 tsp. dehydrated onion
- 4 garlic cloves, minced
- 1 tbsp. extra-virgin olive oil
- 1/2 cup balsamic vinegar, divide equally
- 8 chicken thighs, boneless and skinless
- fresh chopped parsley, for garnish

Instructions:

1. In a small bowl, combine the onion, basil, garlic powder, salt, and pepper.
2. Spread the mixture over the chicken on both sides. Set aside.
3. Pour olive oil into the crockpot and add garlic.
4. Pour in half of the balsamic vinegar.
5. Place chicken on top.
6. Gently pour the remaining balsamic vinegar over the chicken.
7. Cover and cook on high for 3 hours.
8. Sprinkle fresh parsley on top to serve.

Zero Carb Buttery Noodles

Ingredients:

- 7 oz. shirataki noodles
- 2 tbsp. unsalted butter
- 1 tbsp. grated parmesan
- salt
- black pepper
- fresh basil or parsley

Instructions:

1. Drain and rinse the noodles in cold water.
2. Transfer them to a bowl, and cover them with boiling water for 5 minutes.
3. Drain again.
4. In a skillet, melt the butter over medium heat.
5. Add the noodles, and sprinkle in some salt.
6. Sauté for 3-4 minutes until the butter has been absorbed.
7. Add pepper to the task, and garnish with parmesan and basil or parsley.

Zero Carb Bread

Ingredients:

- 3 eggs
- 3 tbsp. cream cheese at room temperature
- 1/4 tsp. baking powder

Instructions:

1. Preheat the oven to 300°F.
2. Separate the yolk from the egg whites.
3. In one bowl, mix the egg yolks, cream cheese, and honey until smooth.
4. In a second bowl, add baking powder to the whites. Beat the whites with the hand mixer at high speed until they are fluffy.
5. Gently fold the egg yolk mixture into the egg white mixture.
6. Continue folding gently but swiftly to avoid melting the mixture. Make sure to not break the egg whites' fluffiness.
7. Spoon about 10-12 rounds of the mixture onto a lightly greased baking sheet.
8. Bake for 18-20 minutes on the middle rack.
9. Broil for a minute or a minute and a half, cooking the top until they become nice and golden brown.

Zero Carb Pizza Crust

Ingredients:

- 10 oz. canned chicken
- 1 oz. grated parmesan cheese
- 1 large egg

Instructions:

1. Drain the canned chicken thoroughly, getting as much moisture out as possible.
2. Spread chicken on a baking sheet lined with a silicone mat.
3. Bake at 350°F for 10 minutes to dry out the chicken.
4. Once it's done, remove it and place it in a mixing bowl. Increase the heat of the oven to 500°F.
5. Add cheese and egg to the bowl with chicken and mix.
6. Pour the mixture onto a baking sheet lined with a silicone mat.
7. Spread thinly. Place parchment paper on top and use a rolling pin to do so.
8. Optional: With a spatula, press in the edges of the crust to create a ridge, to keep any topping from falling off.
9. Bake the crust for 8-10 minutes at 500°F.
10. Remove the crust from the oven.

11. Add desired toppings and bake for another 6-10 minutes at 500°F. Toppings will dictate the final cook time.
12. Remove from the oven and allow to cool for a few minutes.
13. Serve and enjoy.

Zero Carb Breaded Tilapia

Ingredients:

- 2 tilapia fillets, washed and dried with a paper towel
- 2 tbsp. mayonnaise
- 1/4 cup grated Parmesan cheese
- 1/2 tsp. paprika
- 1/2 tsp. black pepper
- 1/2 tsp. garlic powder
- 1/4 tsp. red pepper

Instructions:

1. Put mayonnaise on the tilapia fillets.
2. Season parmesan with paprika, garlic powder, and black and red peppers.
3. Dip mayo-coated fish in cheese mixture, making sure to completely cover.
4. Place on foil and set in the freezer for 5-10 minutes.
5. Heat oil in the frying pan at medium-low heat.
6. Remove fish from the freezer and place in hot oil. Fry until side one is browned and crisp.
7. Flip over and fry until both sides are browned and crisp.
8. Serve and enjoy.

Baked Chicken Breasts

Ingredients:

For the chicken breast:

- 4 chicken breasts, boneless and skinless
- 1 tbsp. olive oil
- 4 cups lukewarm water

For the chicken seasoning blend:

- 1/2 tsp. paprika, sweet or smoked
- 1/4 tsp. salt
- 1/4 tsp. fresh ground pepper
- 1/2 tsp. garlic powder
- 1/8 tsp. pepper
- 1/2 tsp. onion powder
- 1/2 tsp. dried thyme
- 1/2 tsp. dried rosemary
- 1/4 tsp. parsley, dried or fresh, chopped, for garnish

Instructions:

1. Preheat the oven to 425℉.
2. Combine lukewarm water and salt in a large bowl.
3. Add the chicken breasts. Leave for 20 to 30 minutes.
4. In a separate container, combine the dry ingredients of the seasoning blend with a fork.
5. Pour out the salt water. Rinse each chicken breast under cold water. Dry.

6. Place the chicken in a baking dish and rub olive oil all over.
7. Evenly apply seasoning blend over the chicken on all sides.
8. Place in the oven to cook for 22 to 25 minutes. Check if the internal temperature reaches 165°F.
9. Make sure to keep an eye on the breasts, as each piece may cook faster than the rest.
10. Broil the chicken until the top parts are golden.
11. If you want a browned and crispier top, set the oven to broil on high for the final 4 minutes.
12. Transfer to a serving plate to rest for 10 minutes before cutting.
13. Garnish with parsley upon serving.

Baked Salmon

Ingredients:

- 2 salmon fillets
- 6 cups of fresh spinach
- 2 tsp. coconut oil
- 1/4 tsp. garlic powder
- 1/4 tsp. turmeric
- 3 large cloves of garlic
- lemon juice
- salt
- pepper

Instructions:

1. Preheat the oven to 400°F.
2. Line a baking dish with parchment paper.
3. Marinate salmon fillets in lemon juice, coconut oil, garlic powder, turmeric, salt, and pepper.
4. Let it sit for a few minutes. This may also be done the night before to help the juices and flavor get into the salmon.
5. Once the oven is ready, bake the salmon for 15 minutes.

6. Cook some of the garlic in a pan with coconut oil.
7. Add spinach and cook until ready. Season with salt and pepper to taste.
8. Take salmon out of the oven and put spinach beside it.
9. Serve and enjoy.

Baked Turkey Wings

Ingredients:

- 4 pcs. or about 5 lbs. whole turkey wings
- 1 tbsp. olive oil
- salt
- pepper
- 1 tsp. paprika

Instructions:

1. Preheat the oven to 375°F.
2. Use foil to line a baking pan.
3. Remove the wing tips and fat. Separate from the drumette.
4. Place on the rack and drizzle with olive oil.
5. Season with pepper and salt.
6. Roast turkey wings until cooked.
7. Sprinkle paprika over the wings upon serving.

Conclusion

The no-carb/no-sugar diet has become increasingly popular in recent years as people recognize the health risks associated with the overconsumption of refined carbohydrates and sugars. While it can be beneficial in terms of short-term weight loss and glucose management, long-term adherence to this type of lifestyle is not sustainable for most individuals. For one thing, eliminating all carbs or sugars from your diet means missing out on important nutrients that are necessary for good health and well-being. Additionally, a lack of variety can lead to boredom with the diet, making it difficult to stick with.

Even if someone can stay the course and avoid carbs or sugar completely, there are still potential dangers involved. Without sufficient knowledge and understanding of how their body is responding to the extreme changes in macronutrient intake, it may be difficult for them to make wise decisions concerning supplementation. In addition, their metabolism may slow down too much as they continue down this path; this could potentially backfire since any sudden shifts in caloric availability can shock the body into storing fat quickly once carbs or sugar are reintroduced again.

Perhaps most importantly, when trying to adhere strictly to a low-carb/low-sugar diet one will likely feel deprived of energy at times; this is due to limited fuel sources available for their body and brain. Over time this feeling could become so strong that mental and physical exhaustion sets in – not the sort of outcome we want from such an endeavor!

It's clear then that while a no-carb/no-sugar diet might have some benefits, these should be viewed cautiously by those considering taking on such an extreme dietary change. With proper education about nutrition and careful monitoring of progress (both physiological & psychological), it may be possible for some individuals to maintain such a regimen for brief periods but long-term success remains elusive without oversight from specialists in the field who can provide evidence-based advice tailored towards individual needs.

Ultimately we need a balanced approach that meets our daily nutritional requirements while also providing adequate fuel sources—something only achievable when all three macronutrients (fats, proteins & carbohydrates) are consumed regularly together throughout the day!

FAQs and Troubleshooting

Can I drink alcohol on this plan?

Yes, you can, but your choices matter greatly. Stick to low-carb or sugar-free options like dry wines (red or white) and spirits such as vodka, gin, rum, tequila, and whiskey, which contain zero carbs. Avoid sugary mixers, sweet cocktails, beer, or flavored liquors. Instead, mix your spirits with soda water and add a wedge of lime for flavor. Moderation is key, as alcohol can slow your weight loss progress by prioritizing it for energy use over fat.

What if I'm vegetarian or dairy-free?

You can follow this diet with some adjustments. Opt for plant-based protein sources like tofu, tempeh, edamame, seitan (if not gluten-free), and sugar-free protein powders. For fats, include avocado, nuts, seeds, coconut oil, olive oil, and plant-based butter alternatives. Replace conventional dairy with unsweetened almond, cashew, or coconut milk, and explore dairy-free cheeses to complement meals. Pair these choices with non-starchy vegetables to maintain a balanced meal plan.

How do I fix constipation or keto flu symptoms?

To address constipation, increase your intake of fiber-rich greens like spinach, kale, and broccoli. Psyllium husk or chia seeds can also help regulate digestion. For keto flu symptoms (such as fatigue, headaches, or irritability), focus on replenishing electrolytes. Drink bone broth, add more salt to your meals, and consume potassium- and magnesium-rich foods like avocado and dark leafy greens. Staying well-hydrated is essential to relieve both issues.

I hit a weight loss plateau—what now?

If your weight loss stalls, reassess your food choices and portion sizes. Processed "low-carb" foods (like packaged snacks) often contain hidden carbs, so eliminate them. Tighten up portion control, especially for calorie-dense foods like nuts and cheese. Consider incorporating intermittent fasting to break through the plateau and track your food intake to avoid unintentional overconsumption. Staying consistent is key to overcoming plateaus.

How do I handle holidays or social pressure?

Navigating social gatherings can be challenging but manageable. Prepare by eating beforehand so you're less tempted by off-plan foods. Offer to bring your own compliant dishes, like a salad or protein-based appetizer, to ensure you have safe options. Practice boundary scripts, such as, "Thanks for offering, but I'm trying a specific plan right now and feel great sticking to it." Remember, staying firm about your choices doesn't need to come at the expense of enjoying the event.

Can I stay on this diet long-term?

Long-term adherence is possible, but it's important to ensure you're meeting your nutrient needs. You may consider transitioning to a low-carb diet, gradually reintroducing healthy carbs like sweet potatoes, quinoa, or berries in small portions. Cycling carbs can help maintain metabolic flexibility and allow for more variety while still managing weight and health goals. Always prioritize whole, unprocessed foods and monitor how your body responds.

What should I do if I slip up or binge?

A slip-up isn't the end of your progress. Start by drinking water to flush out carbs and stabilize blood sugar. Refocus your next meal on high-protein, low-carb options to reset. Skip the self-criticism; instead, identify what triggered the binge and plan for similar situations. Visualize your progress and remember, one mistake doesn't define your diet. Staying positive and consistent is what matters most.

References and Helpful Links

Ld, L. S. M. R. (2024, March 1). What is a Zero-Carb diet, and what foods can you eat? Healthline.
https://www.healthline.com/nutrition/no-carb-diet

Johnson, J. (2019, December 13). What to know about no-sugar diets.
https://www.medicalnewstoday.com/articles/319991

Whelan, C. (2023, March 20). No-Sugar Diet: 10 tips to get started. Healthline.
https://www.healthline.com/health/food-nutrition/no-sugar-diet

Ms, S. L. (2024, May 4). What is a no sugar diet? Verywell Fit.
https://www.verywellfit.com/what-is-a-no-sugar-diet-2507715

RD, S. B. M. (2019, September 27). No carb no sugar Diet food list. Food Network.
https://www.foodnetwork.com/healthyeats/diets/2019/09/no-carb-no-sugar-diet-food-list

Pflugradt, S., & Adrian825/iStock/GettyImages. (2023, April 10). What you should know about strict No-Carb, No-Sugar diets. Livestrong.com.
https://www.livestrong.com/article/260825-strict-no-carbno-sugar-diets/

Schimelpfening, N. (2024, July 1). Why do I crave sugar and sweets? 4 potential causes. Verywell Mind. https://www.verywellmind.com/why-do-i-crave-carbs-1065212#:~:text=Sugar%20cravings%20are%20often%20caused,hormone%20imbalances%2C%20and%20health%20conditions.

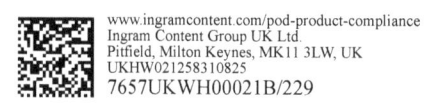